How I Lost Eighty Pounds

And Got Back My Health

Printed in the United States of America

First Printing, 2015

ISBN-1511995521

Cover design by

Dedication

Dedicated to Sean Savoy who inspired me and others to lose weight and get fit.

Contents

Introduction

Over a period of four years I had been slowly but steadily gaining weight. If it had happened quickly, I might have taken action sooner, but because it happened gradually, I was like that famous frog dropped into a pot of cold water that is slowly heated until the frog is cooked.

I had shot up to around 260 pounds which is way too much for someone six feet and one inch tall. I knew that I needed to stop it but kept putting it off. Then during the holiday season from mid December, 2013 to early January 2014 I gained several more pounds and found myself weighing 266 pounds!

That was it. I knew I had to do something quickly. I would have difficulty breathing after a short walk. I had difficulty standing after sitting in the sofa for a few hours watching television. I sometimes had to use a cane to help me stand. I had a lot of pain in my knees which I thought was arthritis but it was just the strain of lifting and carrying all that weight. I was taking two prescription drugs for high blood pressure and still having difficulty keeping it in the normal range. I had to do something and I did. I made changes to my diet. I started exercising. I changed my life style and succeeded in losing over eighty pounds in fourteen months.

I have dieted before with mixed results, but this

time was different in two major ways. One, the amount of weight I needed to lose was more than ever before. Two, I realized that a diet for a few months wasn't the solution, I needed to permanently change my habits.

The rest of this book will detail what I did, but first I must point out that I am not a doctor, nutritionist or fitness expert. I cannot guarantee that what I did will work for you, but I think it will help most people and you can make some adjustments to it to suit yourself. In some areas I recommend things that were not part of my program but which I know work. I also give alternatives to my program for those who wish to do something different.

Eating Plan

If you are anything like me, you have tried a number of diets that had you eating some strange things like watercress sandwiches and drinking grapefruit juice at every meal. Even if these diets worked, you found you couldn't stick to the strange and limited food choices for more than a few weeks.

Even worse, in my opinion anyway, are those diets that have you carefully measuring and weighing everything you eat and drink and carefully counting every calorie. Try doing that when circumstances have you eating in a restaurant or an office cafeteria.

The good news is I didn't do any of that. I didn't eat cabbage soup every day. I don't even own a food scale. And I certainly didn't live on prepackaged diet meals. Of course I did change my eating habits, but without measuring, deprivation or starvation.

The first thing I did was eliminate the junk food. The package of six cupcakes that I would frequently buy at the supermarket were no more! The cookies, pies and cakes were also off the list of allowed foods. Candy and corn chips were the next things to go, although I later started allowing myself a small amount of dark chocolate nearly every day because it lowers blood pressure. I haven't eaten white bread for several years so it was already off the list. Most heavily processed foods were also taken off the list except for rare occasions when I knew I wouldn't have time to prepare a healthy meal from scratch. I also avoid eating red meat, specifically pork and beef. I do eat chicken, turkey and fish, but I eat only white meat or low fat types of fish. An exception is made for salmon which is a fatty fish, but it's healthy fat. Besides, salmon is one of my favorites and you need to eat things you like or you won't stay with it for long.

Enough about what I stopped eating. Let's look at what I do eat. First, I eat a lot of fresh vegetables, usually as salads. My dinner almost always starts with a large salad. The salad should be bigger then the rest of the meal. It is also important to get organic vegetables as much as possible. You can claim all you want to that Genetically modified organisms (GMO) are harmless, but there is plenty of anecdotal evidence that traces their use to dramatic increases in food allergies, obesity and intestinal diseases, so be safe and avoid them.

Along with the salad, I have a serving of meat or seafood or occasionally a vegan meat substitute such as felafel and sometimes a serving of a cooked vegetable. While I don't count calories, I do choose veggies that are relatively low in them. Broccoli, cauliflower, spinach, kale and tomatoes are among the ones I eat regularly. Of course you have to eat what you like. If you can't stand broccoli, don't have it. I avoid potatoes, rice and other starchy vegetables except for the small amounts found in some canned soups.

Desserts for both lunch and dinner is usually fresh fruit, organic when I can find it. Apples, pears, peaches, tangerines and plums are among my favorites. At breakfast I usually have a banana. Yes, I have seen those Facebook posts that tell you to never eat bananas when you are trying to lose weight. That is just nonsense. There is no need to avoid them and good reasons to include them, the main one being that they are an excellent source of potassium.

Other foods that are part of my diet include grains, nuts and cheese. The grains are mostly in bread and I get whole grain or multi-grain varieties whenever possible. I get walnuts and almonds for snacks. For cheeses, I try to get low fat types that are also organic. For beverages, I drink flavored waters, both with and without carbonation. I also drink Kambucha and Kevita drinks because they are fairly low in calories and contain probiotics that aid health and weight loss. I occasionally drink wine or beer, but the beer is limited to light versions while I'm trying to lose weight. I also drink coffee and herb teas. I have mostly been drinking spicy herb teas because they are reputed to increase metabolism, although I have no proof that they work (sometimes things work simply because we believe they will, but we will get into that more in the section on thinking.

In addition to drinking spicy teas, I also add hot sauce to soups and some other foods. Hot sauce made from hot peppers is also believed to increase metabolism. I sometimes use wasabi sauce as well, though I don't know if it increases metabolism; I just like it.

Chia seed is another additive I use frequently. I add it to soups, salads, even sandwiches. They add fiber, but the primary reason to use them when dieting is that they make you feel full while eating less.

For oils, I use extra virgin olive oil or coconut oil. Both of these have health benefits and aid in various ways to help you lose weight.

At this point most diet books will include about 300 pages of meal plans and recipes. I trust that you can prepare meals already so I am just going to give a few examples.

Day One Menu

Breakfast

A small bowl of fresh fruit

Two biscuits

Cheese chunks

Coffee

Lunch

A can of Progresso light soup

A few crackers or a slice of whole grain bread

A glass of water or a fruit drink such as lemonade

Some berries for dessert

Dinner

A four ounce piece of Turkey smoked sausage

About a cup of cooked broccoli with a little butter or olive oil

A large salad topped with Braggs light dressing or Walden Farms no calorie dressing.

A glass of Kombucha

An organic apple

Snack

Half a light beer

A bowl of organic popcorn without butter

Day Two Menu

Breakfast

Banana

Two poached organic eggs on

Two slices of multigrain toast with butter

Two organic turkey sausages

Orange juice

Two or three strawberries

Lunch

A large bowl of salad topped with a cup of low fat cottage

cheese

A Raw Rev 100 snack bar

An organic pear

Ice tea

Dinner

About five ounces of chicken breast chunks with buffalo sauce

A large salad with light dressing

A glass of Kevita brand probiotic drink

An organic apple

Snack

A small glass of wine

A bag of Extend Nutrition crunch (1.1 oz)

Day Three menu

Breakfast

Banana

Greek style organic yogurt with blueberries and organic honey

Multigrain toast with P28 high protein peanut butter

Fresh pineapple chunks /

Organic coffee

Lunch

A sandwich of organic turkey on whole grain sandwich role with spicy mustard and lettuce

Olives or carrot sticks

Assorted fresh melon chunks

Iced tea

Dinner

Two slices of organic margarita pizza extra thin crust

Cucumber slices with Apple cider vinegar

Lemonade sweetened with stevia

Snack

Wine cooler made by mixing two ounces of wine with four ounces of low-calorie margarita mix

A small bowl of Special K chips

Exercise

You really didn't think we could skip this, did you? Seriously dieting and exercise go together like jeans and t-shirts. You can lose weight without exercising,but you will get better results if you do exercises for two main reasons: you will burn more calories and you will lose fat rather than muscle which is what we really mean when we say we want to lose weight.

So what is the best exercise program for losing weight? The one that you will stick to! That's my belief. The most effective exercise in the world won't do you any good if you avoid doing it, so find one that you like,or at least willing to do regularly.

My program has two elements: walking and workouts at a fitness center. I go to the fitness center, or gym, three times a week. That might not be enough for some younger people, but it is for someone in their sixties like me. When I started, my workouts consisted of fifteen minutes on the treadmill, six on an exercise bike and about ten minutes of lifting weights with the machines. It's important that you increase your workout as you progress so I am now doing twenty minutes on the treadmill, eight on the bike or elliptical machine and fifteen minutes lifting weights. I also increase the weight used in each exercise regularly.

For the walking part, I live one block from a park so I often go there, at least when weather permits. I also walk on a treadmill. I had a basic pedometer to keep track of how far I walked, but several months ago I decided to get a fitness monitor that's a little more sophisticated than a pedometer. I chose a Fitbit Zip, a very small and reasonably priced model that attaches to a pocket or belt with a clip. I can't claim that this device is the best available since I haven't bought any others to compare it with, but I am happy with it. I like that my daily results are transmitted to the Fitbit company where I can see it on my Personal Fitbit dashboard. They also award virtual badges when certain goals are reached and let you join groups so you can compare your results with others. I find being in groups and getting the badges helps motivate me to walk every day.

If walking doesn't appeal to you, do something else: jog, swim, ride a bicycle,jump rope,wrestle your partner to the ground. Just do something! My Fitbit doesn't do this, but some of the new fitness monitors including the Apple watch will beep at you if you sit still for more than an hour. If you need that, go for it, but personally I can't stand machines that tell me what to do.

One final item to cover here is stretching. Some people stretch before workouts, some wait until after and others do stretches every day whether they are working out or not. I'm in the last group and I think everyone over age sixty should join this group.

I do stretches just after I get up. The stretches I do come from a book of simplified yoga stretches that I read several years ago. Unfortunately, I don't remember the name of the book. I start by putting my hands over my head with my arms shoulder width apart and stretch like you're reaching for the stars. Hold the position for about ten seconds or a count of twenty. Then move your arms down so they are sticking straight out on each side with the hands pointed down and push the hands away from the body. Then turn the hands up so the palm is facing out and push the hands away from you. Now bend forward and try to touch your toes or the ground just in front of them (Oh come on! You knew that one was going to be in there!). Then come partway back up,bend your knees and put your hands on your knees and pull your stomach in as far as you can. Finally, stand up fully then lean back as far as you can. Put your hands on your lower back or butt for balance. Hold each position for about ten seconds if you can. You may not be able to do some of the stretches correctly at first, but do the best you can. You will get better with practice.

Supplements

I do use some diet supplements when I am trying to lose weight. Just as I have not conducted scientific studies on my food choices, I have done no experiments with these supplements to prove which ones really work and which ones don't. All I can really say is that I Lost weight while taking these products. I can't guarantee that they work and I can't guarantee that I would not have achieved the same results without them.

Garcinia Cambogia - This herbal product is claimed to control appetite and improve metabolism. I take it twice a day.

Green Tea and Green Coffee - both are reputed to aid weight lose by improving metabolism. I add some of each to my morning coffee.

Chia Seed - I already mentioned them in the food section. They add fiber and help control appetite by expanding in the stomach making you feel full.

Bentonite Clay - this is not exactly a supplement, but it is useful when dieting. For most of us, the fat on our bodies holds a lot of toxic chemicals. One way our body protects us from the harm they can do is to store them inside fat cells where they remain generally harmless. When we lose weight, however, those toxins are released into the blood where they can become harmful. Bentonite Clay is one thing you can take to help remove those toxins. I take it about once a week.

Wormwood - this herb is also used primarily to remove toxins from the body. I take it once or twice a month.

Probiotics - Recent research shows that probiotics can be very helpful in loosing weight. First, they aid digestion so your body can use the nutrients in the food you eat more effectively allowing you to eat less and still feel full. Second, having the right kind of bacteria in your digestive system can reduce cravings for sugar and other things you shouldn't eat. Third, you may get diarrhea when you change your eating habits and probiotics can reduce or prevent that. In fact, I have leaned that probiotics are the best natural cure for diarrhea even when you are not trying to lose weight. There are a number of ways to get the right kinds of bacteria into your digestive system. You can eat yogurt, but make sure the label says it has live and active cultures. Personally, I get plain organic yogurt, Greek style when I can find it, and add fresh fruit and little organic honey. Some other foods such as Kimchi and sauerkraut can be used to provide probiotics, as well as beverages like kombucha. If you don't like any of these foods, you can just take a pill.

Vitamins – I don't take any vitamins specifically for weight loss but after losing a lot, I take vitamin A occasionally to improve skin elasticity and minimize the problem of loose skin.

Breathing

What does breathing have to do with losing weight? A lot more than most of us realize! When you breath incorrectly, you slow down your metabolism and make it difficult for your body to digest food properly. While most of us simply assume that we are breathing correctly, experts say that about ninety percent of us don't. The correct way to breathe is to push the stomach out using the diaphragm when we inhale and pull the stomach in and the diaphragm up when we exhale. In addition we should completely fill the lungs when we take a breath, but most of us don't. Most of us take shallow breaths that only fill about half of our lungs.

Here are three breathing exercises you can practice until you get in the habit of doing it correctly. Do one or more of them several times a day.

1) Stand or sit with your back straight and take in a deep breath while pushing the stomach out. Breathe in until the lungs are completely full. Now breath out pulling the stomach in as you do. Take ten or twelve deep breaths this way.

2) This breathing exercise is much like the first, but after you fill the lungs with air, hold for five to ten seconds

before breathing out. After breathing out, hold again for five to ten seconds. Repeat for ten to twelve breaths.

3) This one is also very similar to the first, but after breathing in one time, press a finger on your left nostril to block it, then breath out, then in again. Now block the right nostril and breathe out then in again. Repeat about ten times alternating between blocking the left and right nostril.

4) Stand with your arms over your head shoulder width apart. Push your hands up as hard as you can while also tilted your head back as far as possible. Hold this while taking three deep breaths. Now put your hands together and interlaced the fingers, still above the head. Push up again while bending the head back and hold for three breaths.

I do these four regularly, and a few others occasionally, that should be enough for most people, but if you want to get into proper breathing more deeply, see the reference books listed at the end.

Thinking

Here is a shocker for most people: correct thinking may be the most important part of any successful weight loss or fitness program. How you think affects your ability to lose weight in many ways. One common problem is that you consciously want to lose weight, but somewhere deep in your subconscious mind is a program that says you are fat, you are meant to be fat, you will always be fat. If you have that program running you will have a great deal of difficulty trying to get slim. That program has to be changed or shut off.

Another variation is more general. In this case, you have a goal of losing weight but your subconscious is saying you will fail because you always fail and never complete anything you start. If this program is running in you, it must be modified.

Other variations may be more specific. You may want to lose weight but when you see cake, your subconscious says you love cake, you need cake, you can't give up cake. Instead of cake, your weakness may be cookies or chocolate or french fries or beer. The idea is the same: you crave what you know you shouldn't eat.

Those are the problems, now let's look at solutions. First, it is hard for you to know what your subconscious believes, but it really doesn't matter. What you need to do is start sending it new programming. This is what I do.

When I am walking I will repeat to
myself many times, "I am supposed to be slim and healthy
and I am getting slimmer every day. I'm a hunk and getting
more hunky every day." The exact words are not that
important, use whatever works for you. Talk to you
subconscious as if you were giving a friend a pep talk. Do
not use negative statements like, "I am not meant to be fat."
Re word it as a positive statement such as, "I am meant to
be slim and I will be slim and nothing is going to stop me
from being slim and healthy." I suggest saying slim and
healthy rather than just slim so you won't find yourself
getting a wasting disease.

Do something similar with cravings. If you see a
tempting cake in front of you, start telling yourself that the
cake has no nutritional value, it's just a lot of empty
calories that will make you fatter and sicker. The same can
be done with any craving. I force myself to think in terms
of nutrition.

If I am going to a buffet, I visualize myself
choosing healthy vegetables and lean meats and skipping
the pizza and hamburgers before I even get there. Some
people even go to the extreme of visualizing themselves
getting seriously ill if they eat the cake, hamburgers or
whatever else they are tempted by. Studies have shown that
this kind of visualization can work.

Another way you can use visualization is with your
workouts. If you are not making any progress visualize
yourself doing it before you get to the gym. This really
does work.

You can also increase your motivation to lose

weight with some visualization exercises. Close your eyes and see yourself on a beach getting admiring glances as you walk by. See yourself getting into that dress or pair of jeans that you haven't been able to wear for years and getting excited about it (emotions help make it happen). See yourself at a party getting compliments on how slim and healthy you look. Visualize your doctor complimenting you when you go for a checkup. See yourself doing something you used to love doing, but haven't been able to because of your size. You can do this kind of exercise anywhere and whenever you have a few minutes to kill. For some it might even help to buy something you want to wear but can't until you lose ten pounds. The first time I took the driving test, way back when I was a teen (yes, there were cars back then) I flunked. I didn't try again for over a year. I flunked it again. The next day I bought the new car I had been planning to get anyway. I took the test again a week later and passed. I couldn't let that new car sit unused. Yet on another of my adventures into diet land, I tried buying some expensive jeans two sizes too small. It didn't work that time. I did enjoy bringing a bag full of clothes that were now to large to the Goodwill store so you can try visualizing yourself doing the same. I now think about soon bringing more as I see myself dropping one more waist size.

Essentially its all about developing the will power to say no to the foods and bad habits that are making you fat. Just as regular exercise is needed to grow bigger muscles, exercising your will power regularly will help make it stronger. Practice using it often. If you are an impulse buyer, practice avoiding the impulse to buy. If you tend to waste money,practice thinking carefully before you pull out the credit card. If you give in to your kids,friends or siblings most of the time, practice saying no sometimes and getting them to do what you want to do instead. The more you practice using it,the stronger your will power will be and you will likely enjoy life more when you get to do what you want to instead of always doing what others want. Be careful to not get carried away and become a dictator, though.

Aging

Some of the things that are recommended by experts on aging to slow down that process are also helpful in weight loss and vice versa. One recent news story says that eating too much sugar accelerates aging so reducing your sugar intake will slow down aging as well as helping you lose excess fat. The article also said that regular exercise also slows aging while occasional exercise doesn't. Of course losing weight by itself slows down aging if you're overweight, but with one warning. Losing the weight and keeping it off does slow down aging, but yo-yo losing and gaining makes you age faster. So you should lose weight with a program that is a permanent life style change rather than a temporary one. Get away from the idea of going on a restrictive diet for a few months and then going back to normal eating. If it made you overweight before it will do it again.

Stress

Stress often causes us to over eat or to eat the wrong things, especially emotional stress. Our work causes stress. Traffic causes stress. Money issues cause stress. And on and on. And it is almost impossible to lose weight when we are stressed out. We need to do what we can to reduce the stress. Here are some ways to reduce stress that I have found work, as have many experts on the subject.

If you get stressed out at work, try squeezing a stress ball. You can get them in many shapes. When I was working full-time, I kept a collection of them on my desk. I had an apple, a baseball, a shark, a bull, and others. You can also hang a photo or painting of a nature scene on the wall over your desk and just look at it when you're feeling stressed. Choose one that makes you feel relaxed. A place where you had a relaxing vacation works well.

When I am stressed at home, I might take a walk, do some gardening, or listen to relaxing music. Playing with a pet, playing certain games, meditating, or just taking a few deep breaths are other things that can help. When I really feel stressed, I will go to Steamboat Spa and soak in a tub of geothermal spring water, sometimes followed by a massage. If you don't live in the Reno area you can probably find a spa or massage parlor close by.

Aromatherapy is another way to reduce stress. There are a number of oils you can use for reducing stress.

One that I have used is lavender. Peppermint is another that not only reduces stress, but is reputed to increase metabolism which will help even more in your quest to lose weight. Other popular scents for stress control include frankincense, rose, chamomile and vanilla.

I haven't used them myself, but I found Apps available for my Kindle to control stress and I'm sure they must be available for other devices as well. Related to this are Apps that can help you get to sleep and getting a good night's sleep is important for weight loss.

If you find that you just can't stop stress snacking, stock some relatively harmless snake foods like sugar free candy when you crave something sweet and organic corn chips for when you need something salty. Don't eat these often, especially the candy. Some recent studies indicate that your digestive system is confused by fake sugar and using it often can slow your metabolism. I mostly use the natural sweetener Stevia in coffee and tea and organic honey for sweetening most other things.

Final Word

Hopefully, I have made it obvious by now that a successful weight loss program is more complicated than just eating the right foods. All parts of my program are important so if you you are going to try to copy my success you need to do it all. I have not quite reached my ideal weight, but at the time that I am writing this my total loss is eighty four pounds.

Please note that I do not count the number of calories in each meal or carefully measure everything with measuring cups, spoons or a tape measure. I don't even weight the food on a food scale. Simply by choosing healthy foods that are low in calories and starches is enough.

One final point on when you should check your weight. For years most diet gurus have recommended that you only weigh yourself about once a week. Recently some have started recommending daily weighing and that is what I do. While it is true that daily checks can be frustrating because you will see your weight go down one day and come back up the next. I Still think it should be done so you can notice patterns. In my case, I would lose on weekdays then gain much of it back on the weekend. Once I saw the pattern I was able to fix the problem by making additional changes to the weekend plan.

In response to my recommending organic foods whenever possible some will say that organic foods are too expensive. I disagree. You have to take a more holistic approach and include the costs of medical care that is usually much higher when you eat GMOs and other non organic foods. When you do that you will find that organic is actually less expensive. If you can't find certain foods in the organic section, at least look for the Non-GMO certified label. But the choice is yours. If you don't mind getting sick often, go ahead and eat food that is not labeled organic or Non-GMO.

The subtitle of this book says that I got my health back on this plan, and that is true. I used to get headaches and backache frequently and now I rarely do. I also had sore knees that I thought was caused by arthritis but was really just the strain of lifting all that weight. I already mentioned in the introduction haw my blood pressure was affected.

You may want to look at some aspects of my program in more detail so I will include a list of books and websites to check.

Books and Links

Here are some books and links to web sites that may be useful.

Books

My diet is just an organic variation of the Mediterranean Diet. Here are books on this diet:

- Mediterranean Diet Ultimate Boxed Set
- Mediterranean Diet for Beginners
- The Mediterranean Diet Cook Book

I've found these useful for breathing techniques:
- Jumpstart Your Metabolism by Pam Grout
- The Hindu Yogi Science of Breath by William Walker Atkinson

Books on visualization:
- Visualization Techniques by Ryan Cooper
- Creative Visualization by Shakti Gawain

Aromatherapy and Stress Control:

- Aromatherapy: The complete Guide to using Aromatherapy and Essential Oils by Julia Edwards
- Aromatherapy for Stress & Anxiety by Lauren Singleton
- Stress Management by Richard Carroll
- Stress Management Techniques by Fielding Gray

Links to Useful Web Sites

You can find all kinds of self-help information on http://www.SelfGrowth.com

And for information on healing sounds, try Gary Buchanan's Site: http://sonatherapy.com

For more about me and my personal journey, see my blog *Solar Wind* at http://spiritsun.net

Thank you for reading my book. I hope your got something useful out of it. If you liked it, please let your friends know. You might also consider writing a review on Amazon. You may also wish to consider some of my other books that are available only in electronic format:

Soul Power – Awaken the Dormant Powers of the Soul that lie within

The Best of Solar Wind, A spiritual Blog Volumes I & II -

A selection of the best posts from the first four years of my spiritual blog.

www.ingramcontent.com/pod-product-compliance
Lightning Source LLC
Chambersburg PA
CBHW070938290526
45795CB00003B/1057